A MODERN MEDICAL MIRACLE

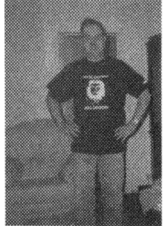

By Anthony Haselton

'One million people commit suicide every year.'
The World Health Organization

All rights reserved, no part of this publication may be reproduced by any means, electronic, mechanical, or photocopying, documentary, film, or otherwise without prior permission of the publisher.

> Published by:
> Chipmunkapublishing
> PO Box 6872
> Brentwood
> Essex
> CM13 1ZT
> United Kingdom

http://www.chipmunkapublishing.com

Copyright © 2007Anthony Haselton

MODERN MEDICAL MIRACLE
PART 1

Brothers, I am born again! And what follows is my testimony, a story of what I believe to be a Christian healing, set against the backdrop of the revival of Everton Football Club in the 1976-77 football season and the infamous rise of the musical punk rock movement.

The blues of Everton were nearing their 100th anniversary, having formed as a methodist church team, St Domingo's, in 1878. They had been an important part of my life since my arrival into this mad world via the bedroom at 130 Legh Street in 1964 as mods and rockers fought on the beaches of Britain and The Beatles were conquering America, bringing a massive swing in cultural and social ways of life both here and over the pond.

At home my dad was teaching me to speak, "Say E-ver-ton". I had no chance, my grandad was even more fanatical in things Everton. Away from the blues he had a ritual with all grandchildren of which I was the fourth. On arrival at Harvey Avenue the baby was duly placed under the sideboard. I repeat, I had no chance!

On the music scene, things were changing. Tony Wilson, a TV reporter, was at the forefront of the burgeoning punk scene in the North West. His influence reached far and wide with his showcasing of the Sex Pistols on the 'So It Goes' music programme. Johnny Lydon, now known as Rotten, was of Irish descent, suffering great prejudice in the London of the seventies. He was an angry young man, lurching forward on stage at Granada studios, spitting out the words, "Get off your arse, I am an antichrist." The song was 'Anarchy in the UK', a chilling warning of the right wing tyranny that the punks were vainly trying to steer England away from. Wilson would lead post punk Manchester bands Joy Division and Happy Mondays to cult hero worship and open one of the greatest night spots in Manchester, The Hacienda, where bands like 808 State, A Certain Ratio and Cabaret Voltaire achieved cult status. Wilson's famous quote was "Oh, to be alive in that glorious dawn", and it was, it really was. I was nearly 13 with the world at my feet. The world was my oyster, but as Paul Weller of The Jam said, "When the world is your oyster and your future's a clam."

The drama of the football and the socially enlightening music scene combined to make it a memorable mind blowing time, particularly considering the events that were about to enfold in my life. Yes, I was born again, and yes I do believe I was, in some mysterious way, touched by the hand of God. That is not to say it has not been a hard life, the lows have matched the highs, but the highs have made the lows worthwhile.

The summer of 1976 was a hot one to say the least, and I had a ball in the endless summer holidays, although I was trying to shake off bad, very bad, and I assure you, I am not soft, headaches, vomiting and loss of balance.

Everton were frustrating, as usual, finishing mid table, but we had signed chirpy Cockney, Andy King, who brightened up the dressing room along with the spirit of the fans who loved his flamboyant style. Excitement was oozing through my veins as the new season approached, despite only going to one game the previous season, a 3-0 win at home to Sheffield United. My enthusiasm for the blues was, however, undimmed.

Most of my afternoons were not spent at Goodison Park, but Vista Park, the home of my local football team, Newton FC of the Mid Cheshire League. The ground had a stand made of corrugated iron with cinders on the terracing. It was situated on the corner of Vista Road and Crow Lane West, behind the Royal British Legion. Many a Monday night was spent at the Legion in my twenties, at what was known as 'Knicker Night'. Unfortunately, the building and the footbal ground were demolished, and a Mental Health centre was built on the corner.

The star of Newton FC was a squat goalscorer, Jackie Kendrick, but my favourites were young midfielder, Bobby Bell and captain and centre half, Kenny Harrison. I had played alongside Kenny for an hour in a training session. That hour did more for my game at centre back than an hour with Bobby Moore would have done. I likened our partnership to Beckenbauer and Moore. Even then

I had a vivid imagination! "Franz" Harrison also eased my coyness when having declined a shower after the game, he scolded light-heartedly, "Why not, have you got two?"

Newton reached the final of the Mid Cheshire League cup that year, to face Milton. A friend and I joined a coachload of supporters to Congleton Town's ground in Cheshire. Newton lost 1-2 despite the noisy support we mustered. A bad goalkeeping error cost Newton the match. Days after, England lost 1-2 to Scotland, a goalkeeping error by Liverpool's Ray Clemence cost England dear. Although the circumstances were similar, the contrast was immeasurable.

The summer holidays ensued. Most days, I would take long, lovely walks on Christies Field with our sheltie, Sandy. Nothing could have been more enjoyable, as we jumped the brook joyfully, Sandy splashing through the mucky water, me falling in probably. The water, my mum said, was full of influence and wee. However, I was returning from our walks drained, absolutely shattered with a severe headache, but life was too good for me to worry about such trivialities. My parents were considerably more concerned.

One regret I have about my schooldays is the chance I missed as a footballer. In the last year at the District C of E primary school, trials for the school football team were held at dinner time, and I could not be bothered getting changed. I am sure I would have made the team if I had. I was a demon left back, with a game modelled on Everton and England star, Ray Wilson, who I had never seen play! My dad and grandad told me how good he was and that when we could afford a cine camera, they would show me films of him. This was the pre video age!

That season, the school team reached the final of the Tom Finney shield and drew 0-0 with Wargrave and shared the shield. I often fantasise about what could have been, that is, scoring the winner in the final. Sweet dreams are made of these!

1970 was a landmark year for me, and it was because I fell in love, with football! My dad taught me to recite Everton's first team to the tune of the Beatles Yellow Submarine: "Number One is Gordon West, number two is Tommy Wright, etc." My three best friends, Billy and the Nuttall brothers Danny and Dennis, who could make the Gallaghers look effeminate, were dyed in the wool Evertonians. We played football all day, every day. Dreaming of playing for Everton and our dads dreaming the same for us.

We were regaled with tales of the legendary 'Dixie' Dean, the world's best ever goalscorer. He scored sixty league goals in one season, a record that will never be beaten unless there is drastic tactical changes in football. The Golden Vision, Alex Young, he was so adored by Evertonians that a play was written around his adoration by Neville

Smith and Gordon Honeycombe. Alex was as graceful as a swan, but suffered with badly blistered feet, such was his delicacy.

The Holy Trinity were the renowned midfield of Harvey, Ball and Kendall, so in tune with each other they were thought to be telepathic, they could find each other in the dark.

In April of that year I witnessed the height of elation when my dad returned from a home match against West Brom. 58,000 crammed into Goodison Park to see Everton win 2-0 and clinch the league title. I shared my fathers joy and boasted to my Liverpool and Manchester United friends at school. Liverpool, Man U, Everton and Arsenal all now shared the record number of titles, seven.

That month, however, was spoiled as the best thing to ever come out of Liverpool, bar Everton, legendary pop group the Beatles split up. In hindsight, it was probably for the best. They did not become rock dinosaurs like The Who and The Rolling Stones.

The icing on the cake came with the World Cup in Mexico. England were among the favourites with an arguably better team than the one that provided the zenith of footballing achievement, winning the World Cup in 1966.

In Guadalaraja, England played the majestic Brazil in one of the best football exhibitions ever. One goal decided the match in favour of Brazil. It was a match made in Heaven as the teams stroked the ball nonchalantly across the pitch. The Brazilians bore exciting exotic names like Pele, Jairzinho, Tostao, Felix and Rivelino. Millions of young English men fell in love with the Brazilians cool, flowing style of football. In Liverpool, the locals had watched Brazil at Goodison Park in the 1966 World Cup. Evertonians reckoned that Everton's style of play from after the signing of Alan Ball following the 1966 World Cup to the 1970 title triumph was reminiscent to the Brazilians.

My parents had a hard upbringing. My dad was an only boy with five lively sisters. My mother was an only child who hardly knew her father, seeing him for the last time when she was three and her mother handed over her father to the military police after he went AWOL from the navy. A few years later my nan took Pat, my mother, to Romiley in Cheshire where Marion, my nan, worked for Miss Yeats, a wealthy doctor's wife. My mum really enjoyed it there, as a solitary child who sat in the house library for hours at a time. This I am sure led to my love of reading. Mum taught me to read through the pages of the Beano, every Friday night from the age of three. That could also explain my strange sense of humour and my exhibitionism at the local hairdressers where my repertoire included 'Lily the Pink', 'Give it to me' and 'Yellow Submarine'.

Dad's mum and dad lived in Derby Street Earlestown. Grandad was to me a friendly funny man who inherited his father's window cleaning round along with brother Freddie. It was later in life I learned Grandad's dark side. Lil, his wife, brought up her six kids with barely a penny to spend as Grandad usually drank his wages. I remember his cheeky laugh, my dad sees him differently although Freddie and Billy taught Eric, my dad, a valuable lesson, how to box. They fought at Earlestown's Blue Pig, where Billy had the ephithet Battler Billy. My dad was an army champion who every Wednesday would push back the furniture in our living room and teach me to stand up for myself, but I avoided fights like the plague. I abbhored violence and used humour and the art of bluff to get out of trouble.

My elder sister Karen shares my black hair and brown eyes, the hair my dad's, the eyes my mum's. Of course we fought like cat and dog, but when she left for Torquay in 1979, I learned how she suffered and fought like a soldier to pass her exams when I was ill in 1977. She now has a good job in the court at Torquay, and lives with Kenny, a Scouser who has one major fault, he's a red! Seriously, he helped me tremendously when I was having a bad time the last time I cracked up, pity about the football!

When Neil Armstrong became the first man to walk on the moon in 1969, my family missed it! We were on holiday in Talacre, North Wales. It was my dad's first holiday, mum had been once before. A couple of months later I started infant school at Patterson street in Earlestown. After enjoying Everton's title win and England and Brazil's world cup campaigns, my dad finally asked the question I longed to hear: "Are you coming to the match?" Naturally I said yes and in October 1970 I went to my first match at home to Derby County. It was a 1-1 draw and I wore my strip in case they wanted me to play! I was hooked and going to the match was my fix. Everton would lift me to incredible heights but they also broke my heart on several occasions. Having said that, in the early seventies I only went on a handful of occasions, and knew every player's name and position. My friends would challenge me to name the first eleven and the reserves. OK, I was an anorak at seven.

At school, I won many friends by helping with their work. I excelled at English. In my first year at the District junior school I finished top in that subject, second overall in the class and third in maths. Proudly, I received an award for my achievements as my parents looked on with pride.

This was 1972, there were two classes in my first year. In the second year, the top half of each class in exam positions formed the A class, the bottom half was the B class. My results in the exams in 1973 were considerably worse, I finished thirteenth in the class.

It was later this year that our school was moved to Patterson Street, not however the aforementioned infant school, but the old Secondary Modern that my parents attended. The old historic Victorian building was tragically demolished and a supermarket built on the grounds. Sacrilege.

At the old building we had a large boys playground. At playtime a roar would arise, "A's versus B's" and a rowdy kick and rush match ensued. In the new building we had a proper grass pitch, where for an hour every week in the games lesson, one class played the other 11 a side. The matches were minor classics and the highpoint of the week.

My spell at junior school was drawing to a close when I celebrated my eleventh birthday in June 1975. A couple of months earlier the school football team had drawn 0-0 in the final of the Tom Finney shield against Wargrave. I did not play because trials for the team were held at dinner time and I could not be bothered getting changed. How I regret it. I could have scored the winner!, well I can dream.

Soon it was my birthday and I went to school disappointed (no present!) but something would be waiting for me on my return from school, I was promised.

The stroll home at four o'clock was at the usual slow pace. I was not expecting too much. The front door was open. I walked in and my parents chorused, "Happy birthday". I shifted my glance from mum to dad, suspiciously wondering where my present was. The answer was in the conservatory, leanto we called it. I walked through the kitchen and there in all it's glory was a purple "Chopper" bicycle. I had not rode a bike before, so I took this fine piece of machinery into the avenue and tried slowly to gain my balance. I moved a few feet before destroying someone's tail light, then I got the hang of it and free wheeled down the slope to the bottom of the avenue and the long busy Queens Drive intersection at the bottom, but I had learned to get going, now how did I stop? I crossed the road where miraculously there was no traffic and my front tyre hit a garden wall, stopping me in my tracks. Now I could ride my new found pride and joy, and decided it was time for tea.

Many new friends were made in my first year at Selwyn Jones High School. My form was 1L4 and contained pupils from a varied mixture of primary schools in Newton-le-Willows.

I had always had two sets of friends as a result of attending primary school in Earlestown at the District school, where all the pupils were from the Earlestown end of town, and 'the Gang' at home. The favourite of my new acquaitances was a well endowed girl from Wargrave. I will not name her but we became good friends. I recall swinging across a brook on a rope swing with her hanging on to my waist. Shades of Tarzan and Jane on Park Road North. Her friends always ask me if I remember her as they assume we were an item. I doubt if anyone will ever be sure except for the girl in question and myself.

1L4 were a great bunch and we had some great laughs in the first few months until my world was turned upside down and inside out when all hell broke loose. There were six of us in the class from the District, Harry Harrison, Fordy, Middy, Tony Hope, and Chris who tragically was killed in a bike accident at 19. There were two big lads from Wargrave Geoff and gentle giant Keith along with Daley and Livvo. Livvo introduced me to the wonders of the Sex Pistols. Two girls sat behind Chris and myself, Carol who was really nice and the gorgeous Janel, who I was tongue tied with. I was in awe of her, but when I worked at Winwick one of the staff was her mother, Hilary, who became a good friend.

It was the first Friday in October 1975, Everton had drawn with Liverpool the previous Saturday and were due to play West Ham at Upton Park in London's East End the following day.

The school day was long and drawn out. Eventually the bell rang for home time and I sauntered down Queens Drive from the posh end to my Wheatley Avenue three up two down council house. I drank a quick cup of coffee, changed out of my uniform and wheeled my bike to the garden wall. First stop was Danny and Dennis Nuttall's. They were walking their greyhounds, while my dad was making the tea. My mam was at work at the Co-op grocery in Crow Lane East.

So, I set off for the school playing fields. They were not there. I decided to ride down Ashton Road towards the Oak Tree pub, singing snippets from the big hit of the time, Queen's Bohemian Rhapsody, 'I don't wanna die', 'Nothing really matters', those words would shortly reverberate in my head for evermore. I crossed at the pelican crossing onto the path over the road, accelerating down the slightly down sloping pavement, gathering pace all the while. At about fifty miles per hour I noticed a builders sign against the wall and a patch of sand. On riding across the sand my front wheel slid sideways, my bike was slipping away from underneath me. I stared hard at the concrete floor below me and face on, I met the floor, like as the sports commentators say, the irresistible force meeting the immovable object. I felt no pain. I felt nothing. The next thing I saw as I vaguely and temporarily regained consciousness was a friend of mine, Carl Goulding, coming out of his driveway and rushing on his little yellow "Chipper" bike to tell my dad what had happened. My dad would be cooking the tea, probably bacon grill and mashed potatoes and watching 'Crossroads'. Meanwhile, God only knows what was happening to me. Death was a distinct possibility. Definitely my mind had passed on to another dimension, my body had switched off to kill the pain, my spirit refused to die. Certainly, I was in a stupor, a kind of limbo state between life and death. Apparently, someone had stopped to give me a drink of water. I had played the role of the Good Samaritan in a school play recently. These kind people, who I will never know, where true, noble Samaritans.

Presently, the ambulance and my dad arrived. I heard the driver say, "Went under a bus, stone dead." He was talking about somebody else, but I wondered if he meant me, for I had left my body, I was falling through the universe, stars, planets and comets speeding past me, I felt a numbed sensation as the universe exploded and I continued falling until the brightest white light shone in my eyes and I woke with a crowd round my bed. I know some time between the numbness and being indignantly woken I was peacefully asleep, so peaceful it was beyond understanding. I heard a call, "Antony!" My mind reeled, a lifetime or maybe a second later, I groaned and an angelic voice enquired, "Antony, where are you, Antony?"

"I don't know. Am I in Heaven?"

"No, are you at home, Antony?"

"No"

"Where are you then?"

"I must be in hospital"

The doctor carried on the interrogation, God only knows what had just transpired, but I knew at that particular moment, I was alive. At that particular moment, I was alive.

When I realised who and where I was, and it took close to forever to do so, I was taken to Hazel's children's ward. I guess I was given painkillers. My mum had arrived when I fully regained consciousness. My parents informed me I resembled a boxer after ten rounds with my hero, Muhammad Ali.

After a while I needed the toilet. I managed to walk there with a woozy head to say the least. On entering the bathroom I espied someone who must have been badly beaten about the face. He had two swollen black eyes, his nose was flat but not broken and his face was covered in blood and scabs. Suddenly, I realised I was looking in the mirror, it was me!

I stayed in hospital overnight. It was my first stay in hospital ever, little was I to know the rest of my life would be spent in and out of the places like a revolving door. I was dying to go back to school to show off my war wounds. My mum and dad made me take the week off school to recover and when I returned the scars had healed. Spoilsports!

When I recovered I played in the school football trials. My legs felt like lead and I did not get selected for the first team squad. Every time I went into a tackle I received a huge jolt inside my head. I kept losing my balance and when we started to do athletics I was last in every race, my time for the 100 metres was 19 seconds which is quite pathetic.

Something was wrong, but the football season was unfolding, I was going to the match regularly. My dad was teaching me to box and I was preparing to join the army cadets and start boxing, when I was 13. My heroes were Londoner John H. Stracey and olympic flyweight Charlie Magri. I had a secret girlfriend and at twelve years old I had the world at my feet, that was, when those awful headaches and violent gut wrenching vomiting attacks were not knocking the stuffing and spirit out of me, although I was to learn that with the strength, support and prayers of my loyal family and wonderful friends nothing could kill my spirit. To those who prayed for me and you know who you are, I can never thank you enough.

I went through Hell in the following months, but I learned, and this thought is for those who have been there or still feel their life is horrible, Hell is a place you have to pass through to reach Heaven, and Heaven will be like falling in love, only a million times better, believe me.
In the summer of 1976 I was a big pop music fan as well as a more than keen Evertonian. My taste in music was liberal. Rock n Roll was probably my favourite but the radio and Radio 1 was my best friend. I could listen for hours. In the seventies the radio played a lot of retro sixties stuff, Motown, Elvis, Beatles and the Stones, alongside Bowie, Rod Stewart and Elton John. I particularly liked one

off artists who had classy tunes but were not chart conscious. Lying In The Arms of Mary, A Horse with No Name, spring to mind.

The first game of the new season was in London. The hot sun was beating down on my bare back as I lay on my front in the dust bowl back garden of ours in Newton-le-Willows in the Northwest of England. The radio was positioned in close proximity to my right ear, broadcasting live commentary from Loftus Road in Shepherds Bush home of Queens Park Rangers of Everton's first game of the new campaign. Everton emerged from the tunnel ready for battle in their all yellow strip with the manufacturers blue diamond stripes down the sleeves.

Leading the line that day was big Bob Latchford, no longer sporting his distinctive beard. Jim Pearson and George Telfer aided him in the forward line, King Dobson and Lyons made up the midfield. Mick Lyons, a rabid Evertonian who watched the blues from the terraces and hitched it to Wembley in 1968, would usually play in the centre of defence but played just in front of Kenyon and McNaught who were the central defensive pairing. David Jones and Mike Bernard, a man who loved a ciggy in the dressing room, were the full backs. Welsh international Dai Davies was in goal.

The window of my bedroom which looked down on the back garden was wide open as my dad decorated the bedroom. A few minutes after the game kicked off the QPR goalkeeper knocked the ball into his own net. "Dad, dad," I shouted up to the window. My dad could not hear, so I ran upstairs to tell him the glad tidings. Two more trips were made upstairs before half time as Bob Latch scored two more goals. In the second half Jones of Everton was sent off and Mike Bernard converted a penalty to complete the scoring, 4-0 to Everton. Wa-hey! My mother returned home from her customary visit to her mother's to a very happy household.

The first home game of the season was attended by over 33,000 spectators including me and my dad and Danny and Dennis. Dennis made a point of screaming hysterically throughout the game and having to be restrained when George Telfer scored Everton's only goal in a score draw. The Nuttalls remained loyal blues, but my best friend Billy committed a heinous crime, he watched the Liverpool and Southampton Charity Shield match at Wembley and defected to the reds. Absolute treason.

My dad and myself accompanied Uncle John and my three year old cousin Darren to the next home game against Aston Villa. Three things I recall vividly about this game. The first I do not know why, but 'You To Me Are Everything' by Liverpool combo The Real Thing was playing when we entered the old Park End of the stadium, and when Darren started to play up he was given a programme and told to read his comic, and Everton lost 2-0.

Life was good in 1976. On Merseyside Everton were consistent in their inconsistency, but I loved them, staying loyal when local rivals Liverpool were about to impose a total domination on English and European football. I went to about four games a season but I intended to make an increase in that number, even perhaps being a season ticket holder one day! It would have to be on the Gwladys Street terrace. Older lads from Newton who were Street Enders were my heroes and role models. I was a fair to middling footballer but I knew I would never play for Everton, but I would shout them to higher things in the bright future.

At school things were so so. I loved English, there was little wrong with my imagination, apart from drifting 'miles away' as I lived in my head so much. I thought the popular Supertramp hit of the time, 'Dreamer', was written for me! All of my life my favourite time of day has been bedtime when I can sleep dream and explore the labyrinth of my supraconscious mind. Dexterity was my problem, my hand to eye co-ordination has always been a problem. Woodwork was a nightmare. My classwork was generally good but occasionally I would drift into a world of my own as a numbness overtook my brain and my stomach went tight with what I thought was merely 'nerves'. When I was reading the words seemed to dance on the page then merge into strange patterns before becoming a blur. My parents were worried, it was clear something was wrong, so it was, "To the doctors, young man."

My doctor then was either one of two Irishmen, Doctor Keiran and Doctor Ward. They inferred I was 'coming the old soldier', and fobbing me off with little blue pills to treat sinusitis, as one crackpot theory went, another was 'growing pains'. My mother was blaming herself, not for my ill health but for her own 'pointless' worrying after being told in broad Irish brogue, "Ah, you worry too much, Mrs Haselton." My appetite was diminishing and about every other meal the contents would be vomited down the toilet. When I had been playing football I would be physically sick and I was fed up with what were now thought to be migraine attacks when I would sob with pain and feel ashamed for being a wimp.

Bob Latchford was scoring regularly for Everton with goals coming from George Telfer alongside him and King and Dobson in midfield. Goals were also coming from Lyons and McNaught in defence, so things were looking good.

At the end of November, on the Sunday after we had lost 0-3 at the Hawthorns, home of West Bromwich Albion, I lay in my pit until 11.30, then rose to breakfast, wash and read the Sunday papers. I was not particularly looking forward to perusing the periodicals as the Toffees had lost, but I was amused as they credited an own goal to "Jack Russel". A dog had invaded the pitch and 'set up' one of Albion's goals.

As a sportsman I read the sport first, then I read the news and weekly scandal. The scandal this week was news of a youth cult that began in London but was now spreading to the provinces.

'Punk Rock' bands like The Sex Pistols, The Clash and The Damned were cited as being revolutionary revolting bands who encouraged violence and spitting at their concerts. They wore torn t-shirts held together by safety pins, with military and kinky bondage gear. The punks expressed a need to be different and individual and have their own identity. With growing unemployment the youths claimed they were being forgotten and ignored by the government, the church, their teachers and their parents. They were being spoonfed lies and propaganda by a right wing press. The bands sang about class war and revolution, cultural rather than bloody, knowing your rights as an individual and not being pigeon holed as useless delinquents by faceless bureaucrats who felt more of a threat from an enemy within than a wider global threat, but weren't the hippies saying the same ten years previously and beatniks and teds a decade before the hippies? Slightly more than ten years previous to the teds the British nation were fighting a war that won freedom for these protestors to air their anti-authoritarian views. Surely there is a pattern emerging here, best expressed in the sixties by The Who, a band who made the seventies punks look like pussycats, in their songs 'My Generation' and 'Won't Get Fooled Again'.

However, in the lull before the storm that was to come, I was politically innocent and unaware, but my consiousness was about to be violently awoken, physically and mentally, revolution was in the air and life was so exciting.

As the illness increasingly took its toll, Kieran and Ward retired and two new Asian doctors, Raza and Nawaz took over. As soon as they saw me in November they sent me to Newton Cottage Hospital for X -Rays and to see specialist Dr White-Jones.

Immediately, when Dr White-Jones saw the resulting X-Rays he wanted me to be admitted to St Helens Hospital for further tests.

Wednesday December 1st 1976 was a pivotal day in my life. Everton had a League Cup 5th round tie at Old Trafford against Manchester United. On the television in the London area, Bill Grundy would be talking to controversial 'punk rock' group The Sex Pistols on the 'Today' evening news programme. Also, there was the small matter of myself going into Peasley Cross, St Helens Hospital, for tests to discover the reason for my severe headaches, violent vomiting and loss of balance.

At ten o'clock in the morning, my dad's sister, Aunty Margeret, came to take me to the hospital in her husband's little blue works van. My mum and Margaret were in the front two seats while I sat amongst the planks of wood, petrol cans and old tyres in the back.

We were introduced to Hazel's children's ward where I had spent the weekend fourteen months before. Margaret and my mum stayed as long as they could, leaving me to have my dinner and settle down. I made friends with a young lad who followed Man U, so there was a bit of banter.

Football is a great conversational ice breaker. It is one of two constants in British society and culture. Football and pop/rock music. They are both dispensable commodities and a great escape from the everyday mundanity of life.

Back to Hazel's ward as evening falls with a fresh fruit salad prepared for us, it was lovely. I could get use to this, but I would be home soon and life would be back to normal. Little was I to know events were about to happen that would change my life forever.

Something altogether strange but pleasant was happening as well. My eyes could not help but notice the shapeliness of the young female nurses and the increased heartbeat when a young lady took my pulse which was probably racing. It was the onset of puberty.

Bedtime came and I was sure of one thing, despite the fruit salad and pretty ladies, I did not want to be where I was. Eventually I dropped off and was awoken at 6.30, too early for my liking.

We had breakfast, coffee, orange juice and weetabix, and a bath. The doctor was called and I was given a thorough examination involving much prodding, poking and protruding. There was a lull of activity on the ward, so I went for a chat with my Man U friend. He told me Everton were lucky, sportingly and in jest, Everton had won 3-0, you beauties! He showed me the back page of the Daily Mirror with a large headline, 'KING ANDY' and a photograph of Andy with a raised fist saluting the crowd. Andy had scored two, the other goal came courtesy of Martin Dobson. When my friend had read the newspaper he gave it to me to read. The front page headline was 'THE FILTH AND THE FURY'. The Sex Pistols, a new rock group, had sworn liberally and conducted a verbal attack on presenter Bill Grundy on the 'Today' evening TV programme. Johnny Rotten, the group's leader, led his group into a defensive riposte to the goading Grundy who hoodwinked them into a profane broadside after the Pistols were plied with ale and bottles of Blue Nun, apparently, in the studio bar. The Sex Pistols and punk rock had arrived, proceeding to shake the staid music industry and apathetic boring British society to the core. One man was so outraged, he put his foot through the TV.

Later that day, I was sent down for an x-ray on my head. When the results came through the following day, a growth was detected possibly on my eye, but

I was required to be transferred to Walton Hospital neurology department for a brain scan.

The ambulance arrived and we were at Walton Hossy, as I called it, just in time for dinner. I wolfed it down, the nurses remarking there was nothing wrong with my appetite. The other children were younger than me, most of them had lost their hair, were very pale and quite poorly.

As I settled in, it was a very relaxing environment, but daunting, not least because, in an enclosed room, some poor child was howling in pain. Later that day the crying stopped, nobody told me, but I knew she was dead, just as I knew as time wore on that most of the children were dying. Naturally, but I denied it, I thought my time may have come.

When my family left, I tried to settle in, the nurses with their scouse wit making me feel at ease, but I was worried. When my parents returned, my Dad was an inspiration with his encouragement and my mum was devastated but kept me smiling through the emotional pain. I kept asking if I could come home, I was particularly missing our dog Sandy.

At leaving time my Dad would say ritually, "Keep your chin up, and don't feel sorry for yourself", inspiring indeed. "You'll soon be home, don't worry," my mum would say, but I had another wonderful friend I knew little about. I was looking in my locker and found a gideons bible. The word calmed me and gave me a mental strength I did not know I had.

Next day, it was time for my brain scan. I was given a general anaesthetic, a hole was drilled just above my forehead and a camera was inserted to take photographs of my brain. Four years later I had another scan for another problem, but they simply took photographs by sliding me under an external x-ray camera, with no anaesthetic needed and not the slightest pain or discomfort. Technology!

The results arrived , and my parents heard the words they dreaded hearing, "Antony has a brain tumour, we will operate in the morning."

Zero hour arrived at 11am December 9th as I was taken down to theatre. I felt an unnerving calmness. The anaesthesia kicked in and an amazing feeling of peace took over. My mum and dad's words were drifting through my numbed but still functioning brain, "You'll soon be home, keep your chin up" and words I had read in gideons bible, "Do not worry, neither be afraid" and "Yea though I walk through the shadow of the valley of darkness, I shall know no fear." From the depth of my being, I heard an angelic whispering of my name getting louder, I was aware of a pain in the back of my head and neck as I awoke from what felt like a heavy night on the ale. My eyes opened after eight hours of brain surgery. Eight hours, my parents and my dad's parents had waited, counting the seconds agonisingly as Richard Jefferies, the finest man to walk this planet bar one, expertly removed a massive tumour.

"Antony, who's this?" asked Mr Jefferies. "My dad," I replied before identifying my other relatives. Nothing wrong with my sight and vision. Mr Jefferies asked me to move my limbs, which I did. Not bad at all. MrJ asked me to squeeze his fingers and with the success of that to squeeze my dad's fingers. I squeezed them tight, my dad guffawed and said: "Go on! Tighter." I squeezed with delight. It was the most moving profound experience of my life. A possible comparison is Adam at the dawn of Eden.

Mr Jefferies declared the operation a miraculous success and the Haselton family released a huge sigh of relief.

My neck muscles had been severed, so I was unable to move my head at all. At regular intervals I would be awkwardly and painfully moved to avoid bedsores. Normally, recovery requires being in bed for at least a week, imagine my families surprise when 48 hours after my op, I was sat upright in a chair, and a day later was tentativelly kicking a tennis ball! Only I know what happened to me then, much of it has been forgotten, but I think I know a miracle when I see one!

My recovery went swimmingly and shortly before Christmas and much to my relief I was discharged and was able to celebrate my Saviours birthday at home.

If I remember rightly, I came home on a Friday night. I went to bed that night feeling an incredible warmth and happiness, but I did not want my bedroom light switched off. In the silence of my room an overwhelming feeling of a strange but beautiful emotion overcame me and I wept with a holy joy.

Saturday morning at home was wonderful. I knocked on my bedroom floor with a cricket bat at 8.30am, the method we had devised to obtain my parents attention. I dared not to contemplate going downstairs on my own, I was still unsteady and disorientated, so it was best if I was chaperoned downstairs.

After a wash and a light breakfast I would have the best seat in the house for my Saturday morning treat. 'Saturday Morning Swap Shop' was a new revolutionary programme on BBC1. Noel Edmonds presented three hours of fun and educational mayhem. Sportsmen, TV and pop stars amongst high profile figures from other walks of life would offer memorabilia and viewers could swap things ie a football for a rugby ball or a telly for a record player. At dinnertime (we were northerners, dinner at twelve, teatime at six), Football Focus would be broadcast, and then I listened to the commentary of Everton's 2-2 draw with Birmingham on the radio. Duncan McKenzie scored two on his debut, alongside Everton's other new signing Bruce Rioch. McKenzie was a flamboyant ball player who played to the crowd, becoming a hero at Goodison. In the new year he showed off his skills to the cameras, but the manager who had signed him, Billy Bingham, was fired as Everton's fortunes looked to be improving.

In to power came Gordon Lee, a man with a Victorian work ethic who preffered hard grafters to McKenzie style showmen. However, Duncan lasted the rest of the season and the whole of the next as my recovery got better and better.

My friends from school would call round in an evening. We would watch Charlies Angels with fresh testosterone coursing through our red blooded veins. I was kindly given first choice. Naturally I chose Farrah Fawcett Majors as my dream date. The lads were buzzing with the new craze sweeping the nation. Punk Rock had arrived, and we were all up for a bit of rebellion, but I could only watch excitedly from the sidelines as I was still a bit delicate. I had a huge lump of unsightly fluid on the back of my head that would need removing after my radium treatment that began in January.

One ordeal I had endured in hossy was a huge skintight plaster being removed from the back of my head, ouch! and about sixty stitches that lay underneath being removed, ouch again!

My radium treatment took place in an old dreary hospital on the Wirral called Clatterbridge. My family were a bit trepidatious as Clatterbridge, unknown to me, had a reputation of being a hospital for the dying.

Every day I had a blood count, a prick in my thumb which was soon resembling a pin cushion. Also, I would be driven to the x-ray department, where I would have my 'war paint' put on. This was coloured lines on my head that would point the radium x-ray to specific parts of my brain. I would lie perfectly still for two minutes on a bed under a big x-ray machine. The highly radioactive room would be tightly sealed while the radium was administered, the doctors and my parents would watch through one way mirrors as this modern medical miracle unfolded before their eyes.

At weekends I would go home to recover from my ordeal, absolutely shattered and looking "like a little rag doll," as my mother put it. My hair was falling out. In hospital, I would wake in the morning with my pillow full of hair, prompting me to have a little weep before composing myself and going for more of the gruelling radium therapy. My hair eventually grew back but it was quite then, but then as a barber I know used to say, "Who wants fat hair?" My new thatch came with liberal rubbings of Bay Rhum.

My radium treatment complete I spent a week or so at home having said a longed for final goodbye or good riddance to Clatterbridge. It was, though, time for a return to Walton in an effort to get rid of the fluid on the back of my head.

The first method to be tried was a lumbar puncture, very painful at the best of times. The idea was to drain the fluid down my spine. I won't name the junior doctor who performed the lumbar puncture. Suffice it to say, it was his first attempt and he was totally incompetent. He inserted a needle in the base of my spine and proceeded to vainly drain the fluid, instead pulling and tormenting the central nervous system that ran down my spine. I yelled in pain and Eileen, a sweet Irish nurse, told me in her wonderful lilting accent to scream the hospital down. My father needed to be physically restrained as he reacted to this virtual act of torture. I still have nightmares today, waking up in a cold sweat.

Everton were making great strides in the FA and league cups. While I was in Clatterbridge I met a lovely girl named Sara. Her dad worked for the printers who produced Everton's programme. One night my parents passed Goodison which was absolutely buzzing. A 50,000 crowd was watching a draw against Bolton in the league cup final first leg semi final. Sara's dad brought me the programme the following night amongst several other programmes from that season, swelling my collection. Everton won the second leg at Burnden Park with a Bob Latchford header. Wembley beckoned!

Almost miraculously my dad managed to get three tickets for the final. One each for my dad and Grandad and one for myself.

On the medical front Mr Jefferies told us I needed an operation to fit a plastic shunt in my head and he had booked the theatre for Friday. "Impossible!" I cried, "It's the final on Saturday." Mr Jefferies looked me sternly in the eye and in grim tones said, "Antony, you must get your priorities right". My heart sank before he added, "We'll do the operation on Monday." I thanked him profusely, I wanted to kiss his feet! Wembley was Heaven to me and a brain operation would not stop me going, thanks to my hero, Richard Jefferies.

I have never been blessed with a children but if I had had a son he would have been christened Richard Jeffrey.

The final at Wembley was a damp squib, a 0-0 draw with Aston Villa. The Wembley experience, the atmosphere of the place was terrific. The seats were long wooden benches that were soon to be replaced, but the highspot of the day was getting the autographs of Mick Buckley and Bruce Rioch who did not play.

Monday was a comedown, back to Walton and back under the knife. The anaesthetist was a young red who snarled at me when I told him I was a blue as I lost consciousness. I do not blame him but what followed was hellish and, I think, led to my depression. A voice in my head kept saying, "I'm having an operation and I am going to wake up" after which I would plead, "No, no, go off into another world." Then my mind would focus on something else until eventually I awoke full of drips and wires before falling asleep again and dreaming of my ambulance ride in 1975.

One day I tentatively felt the back of my head. There was a huge crater! I was told muscle would grow to replace it. The crater is still there.

The final of the League Cup was replayed at Hillsborough in Sheffield, a 1-1 draw. I was still in hossy and Duncan McKenzie said, "Who wants to win a cup on a Wednesay night?"

The Wembley experience could have been repeated. Everton were drawn at home to Derby County in the FA Cup 6th round. My dad dropped my ma off at Walton Hossy and then went to the match. Everton won 2-0! When the BBC sent their end of game report, my dad shouted loudly, "Antony Haselton!" I did not hear him, but it was a grand gesture.

Soon, I was discharged from Walton. Much to my relief, but the staff were super and I will never forget how, along with my wonderful family and friends, they raised my spirits. Theirs and my prayers were answered beyond belief and I thank our Great Redeemer every night for my new life. With all its problems and heartaches, it is a wonderful life.

I asked Mr Jefferies about sport. He said boxing was out of the question, but football was fine. I asked him if I would have to play rugby union at school. "Do you like rugby union?" he asked. I replied in the negative. "I'll give you a card excusing you from rugby then." What a man!

As a child I wanted for nothing, although we were by no means well off. My mum had to return to work when I was discharged and every day, when my dad was out cleaning windows, a neighbour, the wonderful lady Mary Whitty, would keep her eye on me. Like most catholic ladies, in my experience, she was an angel.

Eventually, after Easter, it was time to return to school, but there was one matter left to sort out, the League Cup final! My dad got us tickets in the main stand at Old Trafford, Manchester. Our spec was near the Stretford End, where my sisters and my friend Lynn was stood, getting her ribs bruised. We lost 2-3, but as we walked away from the ground all I could hear was strains of "Everton are back!"

Next stop on the football journey was Maine Road, Manchester, for the FA Cup semi final against Liverpool. King and Latchford missed the game through injury. I watched from the main stand as Liverpool took the lead and rain fell. The sun came out as mercurial McKenzie equalised. The rain returned as Pool regained the lead but the sun shone when Rioch made it 2-2. What followed is a mystery to every Evertonian who witnessed Bryan Hamilton score to give us a return to Wembley. Not so! Clive Thomas, the Welsh referee disallowed it and refused to say why. It was not handball, it was not offside. The blues feeling of nausea was exacerbated when Liverpool won the replay.

On a personal note, I did not attend the replay but at the end of the drawn game, a man stopped my dad and nodded to me asking, "How is he then?". It was Sara's dad. Small world.

It was back to school after Easter. I wore a hat all the time. My friends were very supportive, some clever dicks from another form tried to snatch it off and were duly 'seen to' by my classmates. I was at school part time as I was still weak after the harrowing last few months. In July we broke up for the summer holidays. It was the happiest summer ever. Playing cricket and going on long bike rides on days that seemed endless. My friend Tony and I would lie on our backs on the pavement after dark and marvel at the wonder of the night sky and the magic of the moon and the stars. I wondered at the immensity of the universe, we pondered on our insignificance, we were feeling spaced out. At that eternal moment, nothing really mattered, and we laughed and laughed. Life was good. Life is good.

PART TWO
THE BIG S

Christie's field had been a paradise for us kids, but in 1977 a housing estate sprung up on our eternal playground. My friends and I spent most of that blissful summer playing cricket on the school field or riding through the long winding country roads of Croft and Glazebury on our bikes, but my abiding memory is of our sheltie, Sandy, bounding through the long grass of Christie's field.

In August the football season started. Everton's first game was at home to newly promoted Nottingham Forest. The best manager of the seventies, Brian Clough, and his able assistant, Peter Taylor, had won them promotion. It was my first game as a season ticket holder in the main stand that was built in 1970. The first game of the season was rife with optimism and hopes were high. Midfielder Martin Dobson had a slight injury so he would not be playing. He was an elegant stylish player, only kept out of the England team by the equally elegant Trevor Brooking of West Ham. Imagine my surprise when Martin sat down to watch the match right next to me! Sadly Everton lost 1-3 and lost their midweek game at Arsenal. I watched my mate Martin with pride throughout a memorable season, sat next to Mrs Dobson and her father. Forest signed the best goalkeeper in the country, Peter Shilton, and proceeded to win the championship.

In September I missed the first week back at school as I went to Butlins holiday camp in Pwhelli, North Wales, with a raft of relations and friends and we had a good old time.

I had developed a taste for rock groups like The Jam and The Stranglers, entering a fancy dress contest as Sex Pistol, Sid Vicious. I finished third. On the coach home news broke that Everton had beaten Leicester City 5-1 at Filbert Street. Great stuff! The Blues were unbeaten through November and up to Christmas, when on Boxing Day the players had too much brandy in their Christmas pudding and lost 2-6 to Manchester United at Goodison. Naturally, I suffered some ribbing at school, where I was really enjoying life in 3L2.

I was put in the same class as a Man U fan who had recently lost his mother. The idea was that because we had both had a traumatic experience, we would unknowingly support one another, and we did, famously. In fact, I converted him to Everton! And we would go to matches together in my fourth year as my Dad had not renewed our season tickets. I still went every other Saturday and I achieved an ambition, I was now a bona fide Gwladys Street Ender.

Everton and Liverpool had gone on long unbeaten runs and were leading the title race when they met in October. Everton had not beaten the reds since 1971. An Andy King screamer ignited a grand celebration when Everton won 1-0. I had another holiday in Pwhelli that was superb. I went to my second away match at the Baseball ground in Derby. My first was a visit to Maine Road to watch Everton play Manchester City the previous season.

1979-80 was my last year at school. I was a lapsed anarchist as punk was dying out and I was now a hedonist. Like most fifteen year olds, I lived for pleasure. I loved the football and music. I was watching Everton play all over the country and was heavily engulfed in Liverpool culture. There was a new wave of bands in Liverpool. Echo and the Bunnymen and the Teardrop Explodes released their first albums in 1980. China Crisis and Orchestral Manouevres In The Dark were releasing records that I was buying from Probe records in Liverpool. There were other groups in the scene, with names like Wah! Heat, Pink Military Stand Alone, Dalek I Love You and A Flock of Seagulls, to name but a few. I was in love with life and a local girl who introduced me to the music of David Bowie who had released his 'Scary Monsters' album in 1980. The attraction was only one way, but I was happy with that as I was not into playing happy families yet. I was into Coventry ska band The Specials, a band who sung 'Too Much, Too Young' and 'Stupid Marriage', songs with an anti matrimony stance.

My best friend had an uncle who had two butchers shops in Newton. I started work after school hours, tidying up the window and scrubbing the block. I loved it and when I left school, John, my boss, took me on, on a six month Youth Opportunities

Programme for which I received £23 a week. I was still watching Everton home and away at the onset of 1981, but it was not to be a good year for me. However, in the words of Elvis Costello's big hit of that year, 'It Was A Good Year For The Roses'.

Saturday morning in the latter part of 1980 saw me riding a heavy ancient butcher's bike full of meat in the front basket, and no gears, up Southworth Road to the Bull's Head pub. In the afternoon the shop would close as all the butchers would visit Goodison Park for our Saturday spiritual experience.
The world of work came as a bit of a shock to me. Grown men using the F-word liberally! This also happened in the pubs I was frequenting, notably, Charlie Owens on Cross Lane. Lager was consumed as if it was water. Really, I had no idea what damage it was doing to my mind.

In the September I returned to Pwhelli with my cousin Stuart from Leigh, a gang was soon assembled, about fourteen of us hung out together, a conglomeration of Newton, Leigh, Weaverham, Bristol, Chester and Halifax. There was also a gang from Kirkby who introduced me to the wonders of the Liverpool scene and Laughing Tablets. The bands wrote, 'The sky seems full when you're in the cradle/ the sky will fall and wash your dreams', 'We're in love with beauty, we're in love with wealth/ We're in love with mental health and going crazy', and songs with the titles, 'The 7000 names of Wah!' and 'The Death of Wah!', mind blowing stuff. I would see some of the Kirkby lads at the match, occasionally Gary and Eddie from Kirkby duo, China Crisis, who recorded minor classics, 'Christian', 'King in a Catholic Style' and the brilliant anti racist, 'African and White', among others.

On the evening of December 8th I went to bed having lost my job. Sleep was elusive, for hours I stared at the ceiling with the universe riding a motorbike with flat tyres and ultra powered engines through my delicate porcelain brain, and thinking some rum thoughts. Tears filled my eyes as I thought, or was I dreaming, of the beauty of John Lennon's music, after I had read of his comeback before vainly trying to sleep. Sleep must have crept on me as my radio alarm woke me with the news, 'John Lennon has been assasinated'. It was now December 9th, five years since I was born again after miraculous, meticulous brain surgery. A chill ran down my spine as my life was about to take some strange twists and turns.

With my first wage packet I bought the reggae album by unknown Birmingham band UB40, 'Signing Off'. The cover was a UB40 dolecard, UB40 was the code number of the dole card that was my apparent future when I was thrown on the scrapheap after losing my job. Love was in the air, Everton and my home, Merseyside, were my first loves. I was in love with arty music from Liverpool, and a bit of soul from Dexy's Midnight Runners from the Midlands. My love for Everton cost me dear in terms of work. My militant attitude came to

the fore when I started work at a well-known supermarket in St Helens. My boss was a 21 year old jobsworth who supported the blues. On our mid morning break I tried to engage him in conversation, "Are you going to the match on Saturday?" I asked him.
"Yes," he replied. "But you're not. I've put you down to work." I told him in no uncertain terms that I had every intention of attending the match. He promptly gave me a verbal warning and a written warning was promised if I was insubordinate again. The rebellious revolutionary zeal I was feeling prompted me to tell him firmly what he could do with his job.

Back to the job centre, back to grim reality, and a call from my Auntie Enid on a Friday told me there was a job available at Preston's in Park Road, Wargrave. I enquired by telephone on the Friday evening. The butcher asked if I could make an interview the next day. He was informed it was not possible as Everton were at home to Ipswich. In an astonished response, he asked me if I was serious. I relented and, reluctantly, went for the interview. Everton drew 0-0 and not surprisingly, I did not get the job.

As day followed day and rejection followed rejection, I was losing sleep, losing hope and losing my mind. One Saturday at a cup-tie with Manchester City I experienced the most frightening hallucinations. The day after, I was in a state of paranoid confusion, the sleepless night I had just experienced seemed to last forever, my mind in total chaos. My parents took me to St Helens hospital. I was tripping off my face, drug free, I might add, completely losing the plot. I was put on a section at Eccles ward in Rainhill, rather than the more local Winwick psychiatric hospital, such was the stigma of mental illness. A very small part of the time in Rainhill was hilarious, most of the time it was hell.

The road to recovery was rocky. The football season ended, a long hot summer passed me by and the next season started. Work was found at a local supermarket but my nerves were in shreds. 1982 was a fresh start and was as good as 1981 was bad. A college course started and I was given a placement at a printers in St Helens. When my course ended I was still eligible for another exploitive, slave labour YOP scheme and I started a six month contract at a Newton-le-Willows family printers. To say I enjoyed it was an understatement, I loved it. Steve Martin was a school friend of my friend Dennis. I thought Dennis was funny but Steve had me in stitches, all he had to say to crack me up was, "There were two nuns in a bath". Nick Negus was ten years older but a top bloke. After my stint at Willow Printing, I visited Nick at his new business when I was dumbstruck to hear that he had had a brain tumour removed. He did not know I had suffered in the same way. Months later he tragically passed away, RIP Nick.

The match was still a massive attraction. I had been to Watford and a few other away matches,

Coventry, Blackpool and Leicester spring to mind. My social life was full. I was boozing at the Viaduct club in Earlestown where my Evertonia earned me the nickname Scouser.

In the third round of the FA Cup we drew Newport away. Newport is a rough place and the Everton army had a reputation for being rough and ruthless, not qualities I had at that time. To complete the picture, nearby Cardiff was rougher than Newport and they were at home to Millwall, the hooligans from the East End of London, mad as hatters too. The Cardiff-Millwall game was postponed and both sets of fans descended on Somerton Park, Newport. Somehow, I got out alive.

Into that month we had a home game that we won at home to Watford. It was Dennis' eighteenth birthday bash. To celebrate we ventured to Gossips, the local night spot. There was a gang of girls from Haydock in the venue. Dennis clicked with Ann, Danny clicked with Sandra and I clicked with Kath O'Gara, who I fell deeply in love with. She stood by me when I cracked up in March. Whilst receiving treatment, I worked delivering laundry to the wards, which I carried on doing as a day patient when I was discharged.

As 1983 became 1984 a glorious new era was beginning. I had walked out on Kath. Such was my depression, I did not want to be a burden to her. At the time I was selfish and cruel and I hate myself for the way I left her in the lurch.

On the football front, Everton were on the march to two Wembley finals as they improved with every game. On the music front, I was discovering Pink Floyd and David Bowie. Both artists were fuelling my vivid imagination and taking me on trips through the stellar regions of the universe and my mind.

While I was working on the laundry at Winwick I was turning out for the hospital football team. I had made my debut during my time as a patient. On the coach to the match against Mary Dendy Hospital in Mobberley, Cheshire, I sat next to Rob Rogan, a scouser who watched Everton in the halcyon days of the sixties. He chatted to me in my dazed condition and I was impressed. He was a top bloke.

In the January of 1984 Everton were away at Stoke in the FA Cup third round. I went to the Victoria Ground with about 10,000 Evertonians, and we were really struggling at the time. Manager Howard Kendall's job depended on the result. As he prepared for the game in the Stoke dressing room, Kendal opened a window and told the players to look at all those loyal fans and to win the game for them. It was wonderful motivation, Everton won 2-0.

The blues were also in the Milk Cup, they won the first leg of the semi final at home to Aston Villa. Dennis' brother Danny made one of his rare visits to the match in Birmingham, for the second leg. Everton lost to a Paul Rideout goal, but reached

Wembley for the first time since 1977. It was a very emotional night. To top it all the refreshment hut was releaved of several bottles of shandy which were necked before the drink got stronger back in Earlestown.

Local rivals Liverpool were our opponents at Wembley. Rain fell heavily as the teams played a highly entertaining goalless draw. At the end of the match, 100,000 scousers sang, blues and reds in unison, "Merseyside, Merseyside, Merseyside". The memory brings a tear to the eye. The replay at Maine Road, Manchester, saw the reds win 1-0. At the end of the game, a tearful John Bailey, Everton's Liverpool born left back touched the cup ruefully as he collected his losers medal. The message was clear, "We'll be back."

My friends and myself were stood on the Kippax when Dennis fainted. The crush barriers were fastened into the wall, so I had to climb underneath the bars and fight my way through the heaving crowd to the St Johns ambulance men. "Bring him down," they said. I fought my way back to Dennis, carried him to the front, and Dennis was a big lad, and the St Johns men gave him a glass of water. Returning to my spec, a scouser scolded, "Yer up and down like a blue arsed fly."

The next journey on this incredible trip was to Meadow Lane, Nottingham, home of Notts County, for the quarter final of the FA Cup. There was an open end where we assembled and got soaked, including a Scottish bloke in a kilt and no shirt. Kevin Richardson, playing with a plaster cast on his arm, scored for Everton.

Nigerian John Chiedozie equalised only for courageous Andy Gray to score with what was described as a half volley diving header.

Next on the agenda was the FA Cup semi final at Highbury, home of Arsenal, London, against Southampton. Dennis, myself and Reggie Boyd went down to London, stopping at the services, in the Midlands. Watford were playing Plymouth Argyle at Villa Park, Birmingham. We heard Watford were on the other side of the motorway. We made our way over the bridge to see them. They saw us coming and were petrified. To their astonishment we shook their hands and agreed to meet them in the boozer at Wembley.

The match went into extra time and with about three minutes remaining 'Inchy' Heath headed the winner. The Everton lads on the North Bank invaded the pitch in a state of euphoria. When the whistle blew for full time we invaded again. Some Spurs fans among the Saints in the Clock End ran on and promptly scurried back to the terrace when one or two punches were thrown in self-defence.

On the music scene, The Teardrop Explodes had split and Julian Cope, severely depressed, released his first solo album, 'World Shut Your Mouth'. The Bunnymen released their fourth album, 'Ocean

Rain', spawning their biggest hit, 'The Killing Moon'. Manchester band The Smiths released their first album, that was earning them rave reviews. Songwriters Morrissey and Marr were heralded as the eighties answer to Lennon and McCartney. Late in April, Echo and the Bunnymen organised a Crystal Day in Liverpool including a bicycle ride around Liverpool, a fry up in Brian's cafe and a concert in St George's Hall. I recorded the concert on video off The Tube along with the highlights of the Everton-Southampton semi final. I lent it to the manager of the Pink Pig record shop in Earlestown and never got it back. The cheek of it! Everton played at home to Queen's Park Rangers on Crystal Day, so I spent the afternoon at my place of worship. We won 3-1.

Wembley beckoned in May and we beat Watford 2-0 to win the FA Cup. I was there, I had achieved my lifetime ambition. That was my perfect day. I fantasised before that day of being at Wembley in 1966 the last time Everton won the cup. My dream year was 1969-70, the last time Everton won the league. May 19th 1984 was my perfect day. My perfect year was about to begin. Intoxicating times! Everton qualified to play champions Liverpool at Wembley, fast becoming our second home, in the Charity Shield. Three times at Wembley in a year, unbelievable, and we beat Liverpool 1-0 through a pinball machine goalmouth scramble that ended with a Bruce Grobelaar own goal. The tide was turning and for me life had never been better.

The following Saturday we paraded the FA Cup, the Charity Shield and the FA Youth Cup that we had beat Stoke to win in last year's final, at the first home league game of the new season against Tottenham. We lost 1-4 and there was a feeling of the honeymoon period being over, back to reality, back to the days of struggle and doom and gloom, especially when we travelled in midweek to the Hawthorns in West Bromwich to lose 1-2 to Albion.

The third match was live on TV at Stamford Bridge, Chelsea. Everton played in a grey strip for the cameras. Kevin Richardson scored the winner but there was still a subdued feeling that eased slightly with some good results going into the derby match with Liverpool at Anfield. The last time we had won there in 1970, we had gone on to win the league title. Liverpool were smarting from the Charity Shield defeat and were desperate to win. A Graeme Sharp strike won the game, it was one of the most spectacular goals ever. Euphoria was returning. Leicester were beaten 3-1 at Goodison and we were top of the league. The 'mighty' Manchester United came to Goodison as title rivals and, in what the legendary Joe Mercr described as Everton's finest ninety minutes, wiped the floor with the reds 5-0. The words on everybody's lips were now, "Who can stop Everton on this form!"

The blues by April were in the semi final of the FA Cup and the European Cup-Winners Cup. The first leg in Munich was a 0-0 draw. A clean sheet was just what we wanted but no away goal made for a precarious position in the second leg. Luton were dismissed as we ensured our third consecutive FA Cup final, then came the night of nights at home to Bayern Munich. The worse that could happen, happened, Munich scored first and led at half time, now we needed at least two goals to win in the second half. Howard Kendall told his players to bomb the German defence and the Gwladys Street End would suck the ball into the net. Sharp and Gray scored the goals that gave Everton the lead in a white hot atmosphere. Trevor Steven put the result beyond doubt with the third to place Everton in their first european final amidst scenes of ecstatic jubilation.

In May the league title was won with a 2-0 win over QPR. Another dream had come true. Next, Rotterdam and the final. To my great regret I did not go, but I watched on TV as they outclassed Austrian's Rapid Vienna and won 3-1. Champagne flowed in our house and I thought nothing could match this feeling. Sadly, we lost the FA Cup final through sheer fatigue but as Meatloaf sang in a popular song of the time, 'Two out of three ain't bad.'

1984-85 was a fantastic year for Everton and myself. It was, however, tinged with sadness. I was going to Winwick Hospital every other week for modecate injections that were not only keeping me healthy and sane but were keeping me alive. I was also going to Winwick to play for the football team through 83-84 and I was due to play in the opening fixture of 84-85. There was no greater joy than running around a muddy field chasing a bag of wind for ninety minutes.

My first question to captain George Clark on arrival for the first game was "Where's Rob?," in jovial tones. Everybody who heard the question dropped their jaws and widened their eyes. "You don't know?", one of them offered. I was told he had threw himself off the motorway bridge and killed himself. We won that day for Rob, and played the whole season with his spirit in our hearts as we reached the final of what was nobly named 'The Rob Rogan Cup'.

Rob's indominatable spirit was with us every minute of that final. With the score at 2-2 in extra time we won a free kick on the edge of the box on the left hand side of the pitch. I volunteered to take it and told Paul Larkin to stand on the corner of the area and to make a run to the edge of the six yard box when I raised my hand. The hand was raised as I floated over a cross to the far stick. Paul rushed in, met the ball with the meat of his forehead and into the net. 3-2, we've won the cup! God bless you Rob!

That season was also spent vainly looking for a job. Nobody wants to employ a schizophrenic, so I swallowed my pride and went cap in hand to ask for a job as a day patient at Winwick Hospital. After making enquiries I found myself talking to Jimmy Vernon, the Head Porter, in the mail room. After a brief talk I glanced around the room in a silent pause. On the wall were a collection of newspaper articles about the return of the death penalty. These were put together by chief mail porter Danny Nolan, a rum character who commented about murderers and serial rapists, "They're not fit enough to breathe God's good air."

In the silence, all I could hear was a tick, tick, tick. I asked what it was and he casually informed me it was his pacemaker, then the phone rang. Jimmy asked if I knew where Ward 19 was. I knew the hospital like the back of my hand after working on the laundry, and had spent a few weeks on Ward 19, the male admission ward two years ago. I was sent to collect a sharps box and deliver it to the path lab. This was a test of my mettle and initiative, I reckoned, and I passed with aplomb, I was now gainfully employed.

At the path lab I met Glenda, the receptionist with whom I immediately struck up a wonderful rapport. Another lady I had a wonderful rapport with was the girl of my best friend, Linda Perry. Billy had some strange ideas. As an ex Evertonian, now defected to the other side, he decided he would take Linda to see Everton first now that they were on fire.

Linda loved it and fell in love with Everton, she even bought a season ticket next to me for 84-85!

Linda came to our house to watch the European Cup Final in Brussels between Liverpool and

Italians Juventus. Billy had gone to the match itself. The night was a literal disaster. 39 Italians perished when a wall collapsed and I did not have the heart to make a pass at Linda. The face of football was changing rapidly with each passing season and my life was taking bizarre twist and turns in the same fashion.

Everton started the new season at Leicester and I was there to see Gary Lineker make his debut at his old club's ground at Filbert Street. We lost 1-3, but it turned out to be a most memorable season.

I was now mixing socially with Ian, Neil and Rob who were staff at Winwick and could not care less that I was a patient. I can not tell you what a shot in the arm their friendship was, it made me feel real and ready to take my place in society, although I retained my right to be an individual and myself at the same time. Just a little madness can go a long way! I had a good relationship with all the staff at Winwick and all the patients. It was an enclosed but really happy thriving community. The government, however, did not value happy and thriving communities and were planning the closure of the hospital. I made it my duty to make the patients' voices heard by protesting about the closure, but it fell on deaf ears. I was an angry young man in my punk days and, though I was still politically active, the Thatcher administration had knocked much of the fight out of me. I will always champion the underdog but the Wicked Witch had driven her opposition underground or at least suppressed their protests by branding her opponents as mentally ill with a well thought out media blitz of right wing drivel. Don't believe what you read.

The 1985-86 football season was unfolding eventfully and with great excitement and anticipation. In March Everton and Liverpool were still in the FA Cup and competing for the league title. The derby at Anfield was crucial. Kevin Ratcliffe score the second of the two goals of his career and Gary Lineker made it 2-0 to make the blues favourites for the title.

It was nip and tuck all the way and one night Everton played at Oxford and Liverpool played at Leicester. I went with Dennis to a quiz night at Winwick social club. We were on the same side as Glenda and sexy Rexy, the pathologist. Liverpool won, Everton lost and the pendulum had swung in the reds favour. Everton could not score that night, but I did and a sincere friendship with Glenda was gaining momentum.

For the third year running, Everton had a semi final and, as last year, it was at Villa Park. I went with Woodhead aka Paul Johnson and Sketch. We parked in Birmingham and searched for a pub. An off licence was found and we asked if there was a pub up the road. "Don't go up there," we were informed, "You'll get eaten alive. It's coon country." Civilised racially tolerant Britain in the eighties!

Everton won 2-1, we were at Wembley for the third year running, I had a lovely girlfriend and I was working, slave labour for a pittance, but I was working. Life was getting better and better. Oh and about that pittance, let me tell you, I worked at Winwick for eleven years, during that time we had one pay rise, on our £10 a week, but our hours were slashed, so we were five pence a week worse off. The Tories were having a laugh, the mentally disabled will not speak up for themselves, because no one will take them seriously, but that is no excuse for them being rode roughshod over by heartless bureaucrats.

The Cup Final at Wembley was billed as Lineker v. Rush. The deadly centre forwards would decide the tie, it was thought. Golden Gary scored in the first half and the feeling we were on the road to the double was ecstatic. Disaster struck, Rush got two of Liverpool's three goals in the second half and the party atmosphere of Wembley 84 was soured as bitterness began to creep into the rivals crumbling relationship. Everton were banned from Europe because of the actions of Kopites in Brussels when Everton were on an all time high and ready to dominate the continent. The dream was shattered, it was hard to forgive but we were trying!

It was at this time of the year that a Greek called Christ asked for a penfriend in the Everton programme. Intrigued by his highly biblical name, I began writing to him and a special friendship began to flourish.

Writing to Christ made me realise writing was a strong point in my make up and something I should concentrate on and take up seriously. Before this realisation, I had no confidence or self-esteem, now a little bit of self-belief and self-respect was slowly returning day by day.

The project I chose was writing a potted biography on every Everton player since the Second World War, using my 750 strong collection of Everton programmes. I had a tiny portable typewriter which I used to typeset my literary efforts.

Meanwhile, on the football front, Liverpool had won eleven games on the bounce since Everton had won at Anfield. Everton needed a colossal win over Southampton at Goodison, while Liverpool would have to lose at Stamford Bridge against Chelsea.

News flooded Goodison, when the games started, that Chelsea were beating Liverpool as luck would have it, we believed, and Everton walloped the Saints 6-1. Sadly, we learned that, in fact, Kenny Dalglish had scored to give the reds a 1-0 victory and had won the double. A devastating end to the league season and when hostilities returned in August, the first game was at Wembley against, who else? Liverpool in the Charity Shield.

Billy and I took Linda and Glenda with Liverpool fan Neil Dixon and his girlfriend in a transit van to watch a 1-1 draw, a result that saved a few arguments. It was a great day.

As our first league game beckoned at home to Forest, I received the most exhilarating news. The editor of Everton's programme had agreed to publish my series in every programme of the coming season. I was delighted! Success at last.

My dad went to the Forest game with my grandad who said to my mother that my dad filled up with tears of pride when he opened the match programme, and Everton won 2-0.

Dennis announced he was getting married and moving to Essex with Ann, the girl he met in Jersey in 1984. The wedding was at a small church in Horndon-on-the-Hill in Essex, on the Saturday when Everton needed to beat Manchester City at Goodison to win the league. Saints, the Nuttall families rugby team, were at Wembley the same day. To think Everton could clinch the title and I would not be there… But I would not have missed Dennis's wedding for the world. Football is more important than life and death, but true friendship is worth more than gold.

Fortunately, for my pride and vanity, Everton drew 0-0 with City so the next chance was the Merseyside derby at Anfield. It would have been poetic if we had won the league at the cesspit, but the reds won 1-3. I stood on the Kop with my blue shirt on. The bloke on the turnstiles said to me as I passed through, "Hey you, no singing on our Kop." The amiable scouse humour was not dead, and I defied his orders by singing heartily, "Blue and white Kop. Blue and white Kop."

Next chance to seal the title was Norwich City at Carrow Road. I went down in a car with Liam and Sean, two Irish Evertonians and two of the best friends you could ask for.

Pat Van den Hauwe, Everton's ruthless left back scored after a minute and we held on to win 1-0. We were champions again, cue elation and euphoria, we sang all the way home.

With Dennis now in marital bliss, I went on my own on an Eavesway coach to Wembley for the customary August 1987 Charity Shield game, a 1-0 win over Coventry. I was on a natural high after the game and made friends with Batesy, Cooky and Col. We had a right laugh on the coach home and I started going to the away games with them and Billy's girlfriend, the Lovely Linda, as we all knew but we discovered she was up to no good with a blue from Chester. The day after our suspicions were aroused, Billy rang me to say she was acting strange and she was going to meet a friend from Chester. I put two and two together and mouthed something to my mother to whom I had expressed my doubts. She intimated not to tell him because he would blame me. The day after I came home from work, the telephone rang and I answered. The angry words, "You bastard" were spat venomously in my ear. "Listen to our Billy, he's heartbroken, how could you?" Then the phone was slammed down. I surmised it was Billy's sister, Wendy, getting the wrong end of the stick.

My mother came home, I was upset, and related the events to her. She rang Wendy, gave her the rough side of her tongue and explained my innocence. Wendy apologised profusely and Billy could not stop crying, even though he still maintains I was more upset than him.

One day in April I received a call from Christ. He said he was coming to Liverpool and would I meet him in Lime Street Station? I went and met the Greek guys, Christ and his Liverpool fan friend Helias.We went to Goodison and Anfield, taking lots of photographs. Moreover, I promised Christ I would meet him in Athens. I was trepidacious. I had never been abroad before.

Billy was down in the dumps for a while but one day shines in my memory after the break up. I had bought two tickets for a Bruce Springsteen concert at Bramall Lane in Sheffield. Bruce was awesome and on top form. Billy had always had a way with words and on the way out of the ground he proclaimed his joy eloquently, "It was better than a good shag that." I think he was over Linda with a much brighter outlook after that day. Good on yer, Bruce!

Twelve months on, Everton had experienced a mediocre season. Kendall was long gone, the blues were struggling but they and Liverpool were in the FA Cup semi finals. As luck(?) would have it, Everton were playing Norwich at Villa Park in Birmingham and Liverpool were playing Nottingham Forest at Hillsborough.

Now, in my book, the highest high for a football fan is winning an FA Cup semi final, to set up a day of days at the sporting event of the year, the FA Cup Final. We beat Norwich 1-0. We were at Wembley and we sang deliriously on the bus back to the coach park, bewildered at the sad dejected Evertonians in the street. Something weird was happening. Was I hallucinating, was this a breakdown beginning to unfold? We reached the car park to catch the coach back to Merseyside and bought a Northampton Pink newspaper. "73 so far dead at Hillsborough," the headlines screamed like a siren. What a come down, things were rapidly going horribly wrong. The coaches on the motorway were full of distraught Scousers with their heads in their hands, desperate to know if their brothers' sons or fathers, whatever, were dead. This was a nightmare, I thought, I will wake up in a minute.

We reached Earlestown. I rang my mother first and she said Billy had rang to say he was alive. Thank God. I rang Billy, needless to say he was distraught.

At that time, my Dad's Uncle Freddie was admitted to Winwick with Alzeimers. I spent an hour with him every day.

My mind was in turmoil, I was very confused and a little stressed, but somehow I was coping.

Christ introduced me to his other penfriend, Jane, who I met at her house in Hoylake, on the Wirral. For reasons of my own I selfishly and heartlessly left Glenda for Jane.
Jane was a great girl but no girl deserves an idiot like I was then, least of all Glenda. I trust she is happy without me, she deserves that.

The football season, however, closed poetically with an all Merseyside Cup Final. Simon Pete and myself stayed in Watford YMCA on the Saturday night and Christ came over, selling his stereo to make the trip. In a thrilling match, we lost 2-3. At 0-1 down with five minutes left I departed the ground in a huff, only to hear a huge roar, Everton had equalised!

The game went into extra time as I tried to regain entry, but the stairwells were blocked, resulting in me missing four goals! What a clown! Of course, Christ was devastated, Simon Pete and myself went to the players entrance near the twin towers. The Everton players came out and I shouted to Tony Cottee "Never mind, Tony. You'll get twenty (goals) next season." Tony later said in the press how the Evertonians had spurred him on after the cup final defeat. I like to think I was one of those who encouraged him!

The Hillsborough incident and the other changes in my life, including becoming editor of the Winwick Hospital Magazine, deepened my spirituality and I began reading religious literature of all kinds. There must be more than this fallen world, I thought. Why are we here? What's the point? I had been down this depressing road before and I knew the answer, the truth I was discovering all over again. Jesus exists and God is to be trusted. Hallelujah, say no more. I began to write poetry. Gone was the hedonist, here was the man who wanted to know why the world was the way it was.

Twelve months later, Freddie died.

At the turn of the eighties, Liverpool was the epicentre of the music world. At the dawn of the nineties it was Manchester. I hated the place but there were some great bands coming from there. The Stone Roses, James, The Charlatans, Inspiral Carpets and Anthony Wilson's Happy Mondays fronted by the crazy manic Shaun and Bez. The debt North West culture owes to Wilson is huge. Not only did he bring us the Mondays but also he was manager of seminal post punk giants Joy Division who transformed into New Order. Wilson ran the Hacienda club in Manchester and introduced The Sex Pistols to a teenage television audience on 'So It Goes', a music programme that answered the desperate plea of a youth vainly searching for guidance from a pop world dominated by the Osmonds and The Bay City Rollers. Enter Johnny Rotten. Enter a mouthpiece for the forgotten forsaken youth of bland boring seventies Britain. Thank You, Mr Wilson.

It was a weaker version of Liverpool ten years earlier with a different dress sense, that I was adopting. My friends thought I was on drugs again. I say again because they assumed I was doing drugs when I was acting strange in 1983. They were wrong.

One Wednesday morning I was walking back home from town in my bizarre, baggy gear, probably stoned from listening to the mad sounds I had in my record collection, which now included the Madchester stuff and Pink Floyd, The Doors and Bowie. I stumbled upon Freddie's funeral and decided to pay my respects. I stood at the back of the church. Somehow, that day, the Lord spoke to my heart. I can not put my finger on it, but something deeply spritual happened to me that day, so deep, it was gone from my mind two days later, or so I thought. I summed it up like this. Jesus had been knocking at my door for twenty years, now I was letting him in.

The following Sunday morning I decided to take a walk and found myself coincidentally(?) walking past All Saints Church where I had attended the funeral. I decided to join the congregation and in my heart I asked Jesus to cleanse my soul. I started attending church and bible study groups, but there was a little of the doubting Thomas in me, but I knew the Lord was speaking to me through his word, and I knew I would never be the same again. I had developed a social conscience, one that Rotten and Strummer had stirred in the seventies, but as Bono said in U2's 1991 album, Achtung Baby, 'a conscience can sometimes be a pest'.

After Freddie's death, his brother, my grandad, was admitted to Winwick with the same illness. I took over my job as daily visitor.

In 1991, Billy died. I carried his coffin and read a poem about my Grandad at the funeral. My new found spirituality made me something of a rock for the family who lost Lily, Billy's wife, a month later, but my strength was draining. In September, after neglecting my medication, I cracked up and re entered Winwick. It was a very confusing time. There were times of unbelievable spiritual elation. A deceiving elation that left me flat as a pancake when the exceedingly, heady, intoxicating euphoria wore off.

The year though had its memorable moments. In May after the Cup final, I was confirmed as a Christian in Liverpool Anglican Cathedral, and the very next day, I flew to Athens to stay for a week with Christ, who I now called Christos, and his wonderfully warmhearted family and friends. There is now a part of me that belongs to Greece, but I will always be proud of my English heritage.

The year I cracked up, AD 1991, spawned three particularly classic albums. 'Screamadelica' by Primal Scream, 'Out Of Time' by REM, and 'Achtung Baby' by U2. The following year, was the year of grunge, popularised by Nirvana. My preference was the glam band Suede, whose early single 'The Drowners' was out of this world.

I was still working at the hospital but took a few days off when Christos visited and I made my first visit to Bellefield in West Derby, Everton's training ground and I met the Everton players.

In May Billy hastily got married to a girl called, wait for it, Linda! I was proud to be best man at the wedding in Runcorn. Linda married Billy for his money, the money she thought he had, and Billy married on the rebound. The marriage promised to be a disaster and it was. The worse thing was they had a son who Linda would not let Billy see because of Billy's mental problems that were her fault.

Dennis was doing fine in Essex and Danny and myself would go down for the weekend when Everton were playing in London.

My first visit to Torquay, where my sister lives, was made in 1993 and also another visit to Bellefield. I was enjoying it at Winwick, playing snooker at dinner times with a porter, Ray, who was convinced I was getting my leg over with a pretty young cleaner. Yes, I took her for a drink a few times, but we were never an item.

Mike Walker, formerly manager of Norwich City, took over as Everton boss, succeeding Howard Kendall, and proved to be as much use as a chocolate fireguard. On the last day of the season in 1994, Everton needed to beat Wimbledon at home to stay in the Premier league. My good friends, Rob and Sue, who ran a chippy in Water Street near my home got tickets with me, behind the goal in the Upper Gwladys Street stand. The opposite end had been demolished, the game was a sell out, and many fans who could not gain admission perched in the trees on Stanley Park to watch.

The Wimbledon coach had been torched at a nearby hotel, the night before the game. There was something incendiary in the air that day. Liverpool was buzzing.

In the fifth minute, Anders Limpar inexplicably conceded a penalty. We could not watch as the penalty was converted.

Later, Gary Ablett and Dave Watson went for the same ball and collided. The ball was rolling into the net and in his desperation to clear it, Ablett knocked the ball into the back of the net. It was unbearable. Relegation was now unavoidable. Our worst nightmare had come true.

Before half time Limpar was brought down in the box and Graham Stuart scored from the resultant penalty. Half time, 1-2.

In the second half Barry Horne shot spectacularly into the Gwladys Street net. His shot was a thing of great beauty, a sight of unspeakable joy! 2-2 and all to play for.

We were nearing the end when a misstruck Stuart shot went under Wimbledon keeper Seger's body to make it 3-2 to Everton, Hallelujah! Christos had made the trip over for the game and we met him by coincidence outside the Winslow pub which was soon filled with ecstatic Evertonians. The party moved into town. We returned home late that night, very drunk and very, very happy.

The death of my grandmother, my mum's mum, put Everton's titanic struggle against relegation into perspective. Football is not more important than life or death, five years after Hillsborough, we had soon forgot that.

The Wimbledon game over and the Blues safe, I jetted over to Athens to stay with Christos. While I was over there I attended the European Cup Final between AC Milan and Barcelona. Spaniards Barcelona were beaten 0-4 by the Italians of Milan. Christos and I were stood with the Spaniards singing "Die Barca, die Barca, die Barca, Barca, Barca." It was a night I will never forget, or the night before. I was in the centre of Greece with my pink and blue striped Everton top on, very similar to the AC Milan strip, who the Greeks hate with a passion. Suddenly, a Greek fist was waved in my face as four rough Greeks confronted me, "Bastardo, Italiano". "No, English!" I pleaded pointing to my badge. After two minutes of a heated exchange, the penny finally dropped, "Aaah, English". They shook my hand and my Greek 'friends' were cowering behind a corner.

Another thing that put the Everton situation into perspective was that Linda, Billy's wife, had kicked him out because he had lost his job. Billy now had a son, Karl, who he was so proud of but Linda would not allow Bill access to his son, which led Billy to a nervous breakdown. Linda used Bill's mental illness to reinforce the ban, such is the injustice engendered by this view of mental illness by the public and the authorities. This complaint can now be managed with medication and the sufferer can lead a normal life just like a heart complaint or diabetes can be treated. Sufferers of mental illness should walk with their heads held high.

When I visited Billy in Halton Hospital he was lay in bed staring at the ceiling in a coma. My heart went out to him, but when Danny and Dennis came to see him, we put Billy in a wheelchair and gave him the high speed ride of his life round the corridors. No harm was done, in fact he was recovering in no time. Billy was moved to Walton and Danny and I visited him after a match at nearby Goodison. Danny this time was distraught. We all loved Billy and it hurt us to see him suffer, particularly myself, I had been there myself, it is a very dark, dull place and it is imperative that young people, and old for that matter, look after their mental health.

To Billy's credit he soon fought back after a spell in Winwick, where I resumed the visiting duty I had with Grandad and Freddie.

When I recovered from my tumor I asked God why he had spared me. When I had a breakdown, I consoled myself with the thought that it was God's way of humbling me and my vocation was working with the mentally ill as I had experienced the phenomena first hand.

The next season, Everton were struggling terribly under Mike Walker, the Silver Fox, who had taken over as manager in January and was sacked nine months later. Enter Joe Royle who was hired by Peter Johnson, a business man in charge of Park Hampers who was now chairman despite being a season ticket holder at Anfield. At the time of Joe Royle's appointment, the fans had faith in Johnson, but his standing in their eyes soon changed. However, Joe's first game at Goodison was a derby with Liverpool. Everton were languishing at the bottom of the league and expectations were rock bottom.

Walker had signed Duncan Ferguson on loan from Rangers. Big Dunc was already a favourite with the fans, but when Everton won a corner in the second half against Liverpool at the Gwladys Street End he was about to achieve legendary status. Andy Hinchcliffe corners were already a part of the staple diet of the Evertonian. In Andy's inimitable style he whipped in a corner and up rose Duncan two yards out, to meet the cross with his head and Everton were 1-0 up. In the dying moments of the game Paul Rideout scored to give Everton an emphatic victory and round off a most memorable night for Evertonians.

Duncan was absent from the team when he was obliged to serve a Barlinnie prison sentence for assault on a Raith player in Scotland. Comparisons were made with Tony Kay's imprisonment for crimes he committed before he came to Everton, leaving Evertonians aghast at the injustices against the club.

Whilst serving his porridge, Duncan received sack loads of mail from Evertonians, uniting a solid bond between the great centre forward and his adoring fans. He loved Everton so much he had the club crest tattooed on his arm.

Duncan was doing well but his team were not, though a great cup run was some compensation. Everton reached the semi final, drawn against Tottenham at Elland Road, Leeds. The paper talk was of the 'Dream Final' between Manchester United and Spurs. Everton rewrote the script on the best day of my life. We went to Leeds in two cars, consuming copious amounts of alcohol, even Billy came with us. On arrival in Leeds we mingled with the Cockneys and enjoyed some friendly banter with them.

In the ground, Everton had three sides of the ground, with Spurs in the huge new stand. It proved to our advantage, the atmosphere was electric as Everton dominated and took the lead with a Matt Jackson near post header from a trademark Hinchcliffe corner. Graham Stuart made it 2-0 in the second half, then Spurs won a dubious penalty that Jurgen Klinnsman, the German striker, scored. This served only to galvanise Everton. Their play was vintage School of Science stuff. Rideout went down injured and Daniel Amokachi, unknown to his manager, entered the field of play, scoring two blinders to give Everton a crushing 4-1 victory. Joe Royle said it was the best substitution he had never made, and made no apologies for spoiling the 'Dream Final'.

Manchester United were hot favourites for the final at Wembley. If the semi final had been the best day of my life, Wembley '95 was the best weekend. I went down to Dennis's in Horndon-on-the-Hill, or Hardon-on-the-Hill as Dennis called it, on the Friday. We went for a bevvy on the Friday night to local hostelries, 'The Bell' and 'The Swan'. On the stagger back to Dennis' house, a black cat crossed our path, a confidence boosting piece of folklore indeed.

Three of us made the trip to Wembley by train. Dennis, myself and Colin, an ex-policeman from Newton-le-Willows, whom Dennis had met in Essex by pure coincidence. It was a fantastic atmosphere, particularly outside the stadium before the game, my cup ranneth over.

It was a poor game but Everton won by a Paul Rideout header to nil, and the celebrations were intoxicating as we reclaimed United's song to rub it in, 'Always Look On The Bright Side Of Life'.

On the Sunday, with a bleary head, I bought all the Sunday newspapers and boarded the Liverpool train from Euston with one bag of newspapers in one hand, and a bag of clothes in the other.

Arriving in Liverpool was magic. It was the first occasion I had entered Lime Street from the London direction and beholding the three graces was a wonderful homecoming. As the Evertonians walked up the concourse at the station, we were applauded by the Liverpool public as if we were players. I felt like a hero returning from the war, ten feet tall, fantastic!

It was about one o'clock, so I rang home to tell my ma that I would not be home yet, as I was going to Walton to watch the open top bus homecoming. So, bags in hand I boarded the bus to Walton and watched the victorious team parade the chalice of the Holy Grail through the streets of Liverpool.

Reflecting on the glory of the weekend as I travelled home on the train, I felt on top of the world, looking down on creation, if I may quote Karen Carpenter. The breakdowns were merely a blip. The triumphs I shared with all my super Everton friends, as well as the many heartaches we shared, were the sunshine after the rain and in a funny kind of way a little miracle, not least for making the battles worth fighting through and giving the assurance that the battle of life is worth fighting, for the rewards of a certain victory are the wonderful prize of life, love, joy and peace, by the bucketful.

My parents split up in 1983 when my mum kicked my dad out, after he 'wandered'. A miracle occurred in 1995. They were still friends. My dad moved into my nan's vacant house after a big bust up with his girlfriend. My mum's visits became more frequent, so my sister and I encouraged mum to 'court' my dad. Soon, she was staying weekends and in the summer of '95 my parents and I travelled to Karen's home in Torquay, staying for a week, although my dad stayed in a guest house, while Mum and I stayed at Kenny and Karen's in Plainmoor, near the football ground of the same name.

I discovered a groovy watering hole called The Piazza where two bands played during my stay. A band called Whiteout played there on the Sunday. I had never heard of them, but I was well impressed, duly buying their flop but brilliant CD 'Bite It'.

On the Monday, there was a tribute band playing in the Piazza named 'The Resurrection of The Doors'. They played cover versions of Doors songs, and sounded just like the originals. Fuelled by alcohol, I danced wildly with a dream of a girl, who disappeared into the night. Imagine my surprise when, in a supermarket queue, I came face to face with the angelic apparition that was Jenny. I asked her out, but she politely declined my offer. It was not to be, but she made my week, with The Doors and Whiteout, that is. To top it all my Dad moved back home the following year.

Everton's attempt to secure the signature of Andrei Kanchelskis from Manchester United was turning into a saga. Eventually he was signed but a local United fan told me that he would do the dirty on Everton just as he had done on United. Apparently, Andrei was a heavy gambler and loyalty was not a word in the Ukrainean's English vocabulary.

The blues played some excellent football with Andrei performing brilliantly down the right wing and Swede Anders Limpar down the left. Everton narrowly missed out on European qualification in the league but visited Iceland and Holland in the European Cup Winners Cup.

Rumours had been circulating around Winwick Hospital for years about its closure, but in 1996 it was enforced. The run down was immediate as ward by ward the demise of the great institution ensued.

There was one plus point for me, personally. The corridor that the library was on was closed. I was based in the library which remained open. The empty wards were used as film sets for local television companies. Edward Woodward's 'In Suspicious Circumstances' was filmed there and I met the man himself, serving him, the other actors and film crew with tea and biscuits in the library. In fact, a gallows was built in a courtyard for one scene. Gruesome!

A play called 'The Beat Goes On' was also filmed there. As the hospitals roving reporter, I had the honour of being the only member of staff allowed to wander the film set. I interviewed Jenny Agutter (famous for her role in 'The Railway Children') and John McArdle, better known as Billy Corkhill of Brookside.

My love life blossmed as well that spring. I had a fling with the Lovely Linda from Widnes. Our favourite record was 'Astral Weeks' by Van Morrison. One of the tracks was 'Cyprus Avenue'. By coincidence I visited Linda's home in, yes, Cypress Avenue, only the spelling changed.

Christmas 1996 drew a veil over my working life at Winwick. The library closed and I was out of a job. Everton's form was patchy with Kanchelskis a shadow of the previous season's flyer, but when Everton beat Derby at the Baseball Ground at Christmas, with a late Nick Barmby goal, they were tipped as dark horses for the title. Unfortunately, the Toffee's form went rapidly downhill. They were beaten by bottom of the league Nottingham Forest at home and that was devastating, exacerbated by an inspired lob from first division Bradford's England international Chris Waddle in their elimination of Everton from the FA Cup.

Joe Royle did not get the support of his chairman at this difficult time and resigned. The fans turned on Johnson and demanded his departure from the club, but Johnson stood firm despite the hatred.

Everton struggled to stay in the Premier League as form plunged dramatically, Dave Watson doing a sterling job as caretaker manager before Howard Kendall returned to the fray for the third time as manager.

Days were dark and dull at Goodison, as mediocre players joined the club and fortunes plunged. Speaking of fortunes, the fans demanded angrily of Johnson, "Where's the money?"

I developed a hernia and went into St Helens Hospital for an operation. By this time my father had returned home. I was no longer man of the house. Whilst I was in hospital, Everton were beaten 1-4 at Coventry in a league cup match. At the end there was bust up betweem Kendall and defender Craig Short. All the lads on the ward took the micky, but it insured I did not feel sorry for myself. I had to laugh it off, which aided my recovery. Laughter really is the finest medicine.

In September, mum and dad went on holiday while I stayed at home to look after the cats, Bonnie, a beautiful fiercely independent tortoiseshell, and Suki, a Persian, black and white with no tail. She was in a tragically sorry state when a customer of my dad's found her cowering in her garage. My dad rescued her, she now lives contentedly at home with the Haselton family in Wheatley Avenue.

On the Sunday when my parents were away I rose to read the headlines 'Di Battles For Life'. I immediately put on the TV, and I heard the chilling words, 'Princess Di is dead'. I had her photograph on my wall at work, I admired her looks and her grace and genuine compassion, and she was dead. I went to church hoping to find some solace but I heard in the service the news of the recent death of Janice Glynn, apparently from lupus. Janice was a nurse at Winwick and a dear friend who often gave me a lift to work. With the news of the death of two women I thought highly of, I returned to an empty house. I was so low, it was awful. The feeling was exacerbated when a particularly grey day I got wet through and caught a bug. It was a terrible virus that was doing the rounds and I consequently felt like death. As Christmas approached with its commercial glitz and accompanying pressure, my depression deepened. On Boxing Day I cracked up and ended up in Winwick after a nightmare Christmas.

Like a rubberball I bounced back again, enjoying a friendship with Julie Jones who worked at Market Chambers, a drop in centre for people in Newton and Haydock who could not work because of mental problems. I went there after a regular appointment with my psychiatrist. I had told her that I had tried to work, at Warrington Market and at Industrial Therapy at Winwick. Now my chemicals and hormones were upside down, I was anxious about my future, I was flipping bored to tears, almost literally, and I wanted a job!

I was told there were no jobs, but she recommended Market Chambers to occupy my time.

Julie J was great fun and aided my recovery remarkably, along with the other users of the centre and the rest of the staff. JJ and I went to Liverpool to watch Casablanca at the ABC as the last film to show there as the cinema was to close. The entry fee was a pound! The response was tremendous. At the time I was off my head as I was going through an experimental phase with my medication. I was buzzing with adrenalin.

On one of my frequent visits to Liverpool, I now had a train pass and was getting the most out of it, I picked up an Echo and read an advertisement for a course at Liverpool Institute of Performing Arts, LIPA for short. I undertook a ten week course training disabled artists to run workshops. It was really, really interesting and we did all kind of weird and wonderful exercises. The others who were on the course were all brilliant, very talented and all had physical disabilities and all were truly inspiring. When it came round to placement time I lost my bottle and packed it in. I was not a hundred per cent yet, although I sold a few copies of 'A Sense Of Perception', a book I contributed ten poems to and a biography of myself. I was given the title 'A Spotlight Poet' and I was proud of myself, but I have always had the feeling I could do more and must keep pushing back the parameters of experience and imagination.

Visits had been made to Athens in 1997 and 2000. I love Greece. I recall visiting the Acropolis alone, Christos did not have the admission fee, and I surveyed the city thinking, this is me!, this is Tony at the Acropolis, mind blowing!

Now, we were in a new century and a new millennium but little had changed, then again if someone had said I would stand at the Acropolis, a published poet in 1983, I would have laughed. I am only telling this story to illustrate schizophrenia need not stop personal development. Dreams can come true, so don't lose your dreams.

The aftercare I received on discharge from Winwick in 1997 was excellent. Labour were now in power reinforcing my dislike of the Tory administration I felt had ruined my life.

Two years after a wonderful week in Lanzarote, where I had the pleasure of being hypnotised, I was invited to Officespace in St Helens for an interview. It was a factory specialising in the upkeep of horse blankets known as Workspace, but in 2001 they started Officespace in the same building where people with mental problems could be trained for office work. It was a wise move. My confidence boomed. One of the benefits of it was two weekend breaks at the Norbreck Castle Hotel in Blackpool. It was a top class hotel with jacuzzis, steam rooms and lovely food. Nice!

I had started going to the match with a bloke called Roy and I asked him to accompany me on Everton's pre-season tour of Devon. We stayed at Karen's and we attended games at St James Park in Exeter and Home Park in Plymouth. Huish Park in Yeovil proved too difficult to get to.

2002 saw me jobless again, but I was enjoying the company of new found friends at Market Chambers, which like Winwick before it, was a fine useful place that was earmarked for closure. We were promised alternative premises would be found. In 2003 MC closed for good. As they say in politics, a lie is a lie is a lie.

On a Friday I attended a men's group. To my great surprise, an old neighbour started attending. I became good friends with Paul and we holidayed in Tenerife together and had a great week despite me losing my money which was found in an undiscovered 'secret' pocket in my bag, on return to base in Newton, much to my embarrassment.

In August of that year, I journeyed to Wrexham in North Wales to watch Everton in a pre-season friendly. A sixteen year old named Wayne Rooney made his debut. A few weeks later, Everton, now under the management of David Moyes, were at home to Arsenal. The London team had gone over twelve months without a defeat. As reigning champions it looked certain they were going to extend that run when they took the lead at Goodison where I was watching from the Bullens Road stand. Surprisingly Radzinski equalised, Rooney came on as substitute and with the game nearing the end he received the ball thirty yards from goal. With little back swing he chipped the ball over the head of England's keeper David Seaman and under the crossbar. Everton won 2-1! On the TV the commentator said: "Remember where you heard the name first, Wayne Rooney!"

After a good season for Everton, narrowly missing out on a European place, I travelled with Paul to Zakynthos, otherwise known as Zante in Greece, by which time I was seeing Annette whom I had met at a New Year's Eve party at the Sunbeam, which became the local for our social group.

Thanks to Dave Sweeney and Jackie Hill, two health service professionals and good friends, I became a member of St Helens Mental Health

Promotion Team, working for Dave, an ex-punk rocker who now has a top job for the Primary Care Trust. We were visiting work places giving talks about good mental health, stressing that good mental health was for everyone, not just those with an illness. It is shocking the misconceptions the general public have of mental illness.

In 2005 I began writing the story you are reading now, after making a two minute film for the BBC on the same subject. I appeared in a play that we are still being asked to perform. It is about dual diagnosis, the combined problem of mental illness and a drink/drug problem. Jackie, Gill Keight and myself are spreading the word around the North West about good mental health via talks to work places. I have fifteen minutes telling my story, and it gives me a real buzz.

Depression knocks at my door still, but the door is firmly bolted. There is help for the mentally ill. If you encounter it, say loudly:

I MAY BE MAD
BUT I AM AT PEACE
I HAVE NOTHING TO PROVE
TO AN IGNORANT WORLD
AND I HOLD MY HEAD HIGH.

www.ingramcontent.com/pod-product-compliance
Lightning Source LLC
Chambersburg PA
CBHW031928080426
42734CB00007B/599